Show your FOOD who's BOSS

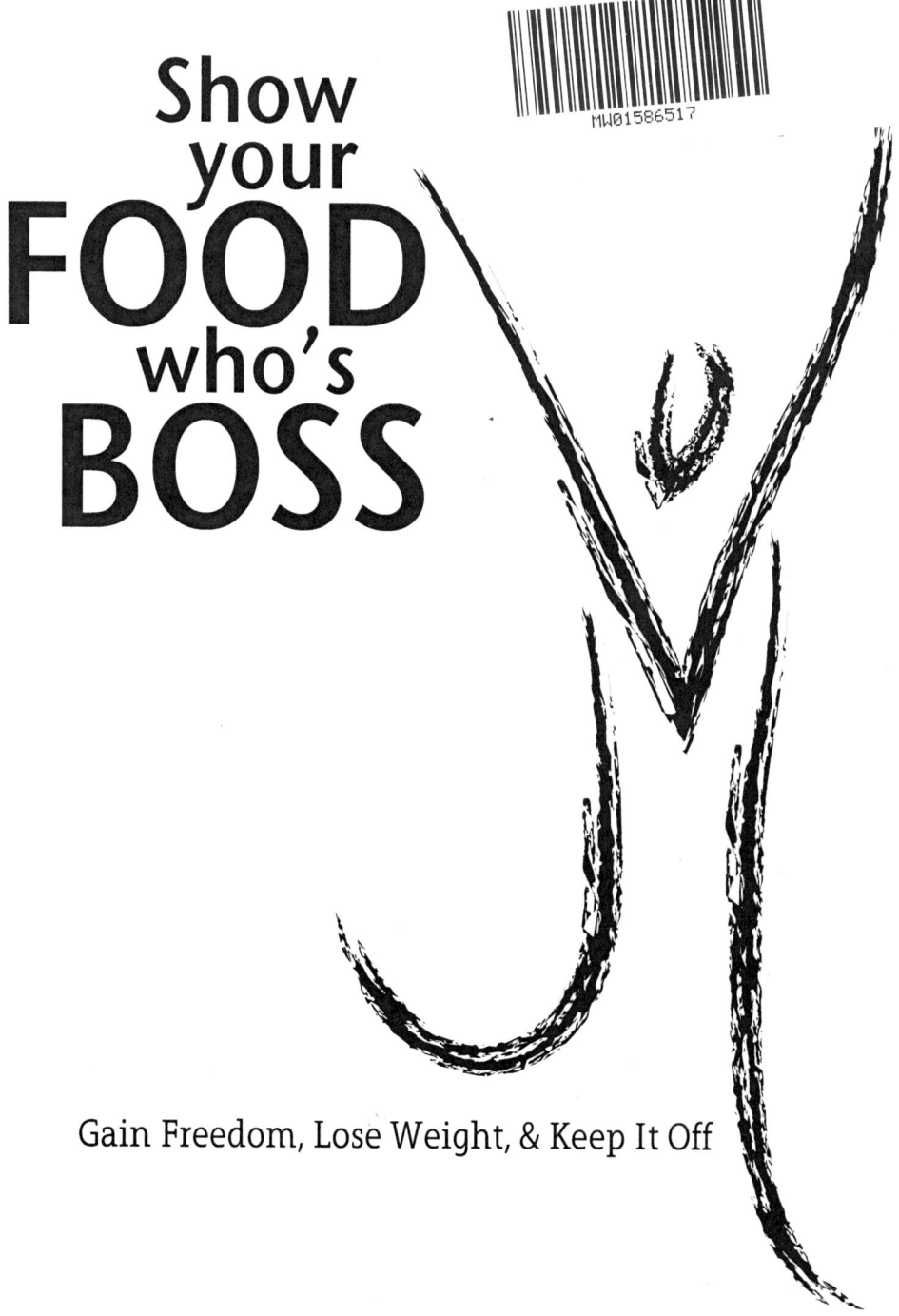

Gain Freedom, Lose Weight, & Keep It Off

Mary Lou Caskey
www.maryloucaskey.com

Show Your Food Who's Boss:
Gain Freedom, Lose Weight, & Keep it Off

Copyright © 2013 by Mary Lou Caskey

Published by Mary Lou Caskey
www.maryloucaskey.com

Unless otherwise indicated, all Scripture quotations are taken from the Holy Bible, New Living Translation, copyright © 1996, 2004, 2007 by Tyndale House Foundation. Used by permission of Tyndale House Publishers, Inc., Carol Stream, Illinois 60188. All rights reserved.

Verses marked with NIV are taken from the NEW INTERNATIONAL VERSION®. NIV®. Copyright © 1973, 1978, 1984 by the International Bible Society. Used by permission of Zondervan. All rights reserved.

Verses marked with MSG are taken from The Message. Copyright © Eugene H. Peterson 1993, 1994, 1995, 1996, 2000, 2001, 2002. Used by permission of NavPress Publishing Group.

Cover by iBloom – http://ibloom.us

ISBN: 978-0-9826626-6-3

All rights reserved. No part of this publication may be reproduced, stored in a removal system, or transmitted in any form or by any means – electronic, mechanical, digital, photocopy, recording, or any other – except for brief quotations in printed reviews, without the prior permission of the publisher.

This book is not intended to provide counseling, clinical advice, or take the place of treatment from your personal physician or professional mental health provider. Readers are advised to consult their own qualified health-care physicians regarding mental health and medical issues. Neither the publisher nor the author takes any responsibility for any possible consequences from actions or application of information in this book to reader.

To anyone who has ever struggled with food or weight,
my prayer for you...

"When I think of all this, I fall to my knees and pray to the Father, the Creator of everything in heaven and on earth. I pray that from his glorious, unlimited resources he will empower you with inner strength through his Spirit. Then Christ will make his home in your hearts as you trust in him. Your roots will grow down into God's love and keep you strong. And may you have the power to understand, as all God's people should, how wide, how long, how high, and how deep his love is. May you experience the love of Christ, though it is too great to understand fully. Then you will be made complete with all the fullness of life and power that comes from God.

Now all glory to God, who is able, through his mighty power at work within us, to accomplish infinitely more than we might ask or think." **Ephesians 3:14-20**

Acknowledgements

God, words won't begin to express how grateful I am for what you have done in my life. Thank you also for the opportunities to make a difference in the lives of others.

Keith, your unconditional love and support is such a gift in my life. You help me to be a better person. I am blessed to have the privilege of being married to you.

Dad and Mom, thank you for how you love our entire family so well. I am grateful for you.

Rachel and Noel, you are both such incredible, courageous, hard working and determined women. I work hard to grow personally because of both of you and Keanu, Ayden, Ricky and RG.

New Life Ministries, Steve Arterburn and team, thank you for the major impact you've had on my life.

iBloom – Kelly Thorne Gore and team, thank you for all of your work on this project. It would never have happened without you.

There are so many people that I want to thank, but I would not be able to name everyone who has impacted my life to this point.

Thank you also to so many people who have prayed for me through this project, have given input and have listened to me. I am grateful!
Thank you.

Contents

Introduction	8
1. Find Your Own "Why"	11
2. One Size Does NOT Fit All	17
3. Adventure Buddies	23
4. Set Goals That Work For You	31
5. Empower or Backfire	37
6. I'm Stressed! Who Has the Chocolate?	42
7. Food is No Longer Center Stage	53
8. A New and Easier Relationship with Food	60
9. Weight Loss Is a Sensitive Subject	69
10. Spiritual Renewal and Empowerment	82
11. Group Discussion	109
Conclusion	123
References	125

Scan this QR code using your smart phone or go to www.maryloucaskey.com/free-gift to get my free gift for you!

Introduction

As a child I was ridiculed and bullied for my size even though I was only chubby. I really didn't think about my size and didn't try to lose weight until I was in my mid 20's.

I gained a healthy amount of weight during my first pregnancy and quickly was able to lose the weight and get back into my regular clothes. During my second pregnancy, I gained a lot of weight, and this time, I was eight sizes larger than I had ever been in my life. I didn't know what to do. It was the first time in my life that I looked for a weight loss solution. That was the beginning of the 20 years of the "weight loss process yo-yo" for me. I tried almost everything that was available during those years. You may relate to trying everything and hoping each time, saying to yourself, "This is it!"

I was tired of the yo-yo. I desired lasting change, but something was missing. There had to be something I wasn't considering or incorporating. I just didn't know what it was!

The good news is that I discovered the missing pieces that were sabotaging my ability to lose weight and keep it off. I didn't have a "formulated plan" that I followed from start to finish. Rather, I learned how to "do the next right thing." Each phase of my adventure provided something new for me to implement. The process of losing weight provided me the greatest potential for spiritual and personal growth, and I believe it can do the same for you. I am very grateful that I not only lost the weight, but I have also kept it off for years. What means even more to me is that I am now at peace with food and I am passionate about helping others gain freedom. Peace with food to me means that I simply enjoy food; it no longer has power over me. I can go anywhere I want and barely notice the food that is there. I'm not spending any energy on yo-yo dieting, which brings me freedom in many areas of life. I am so grateful to be free from those constraints for the rest of my life.

Creating lasting change in any area of life can be challenging, but the good news is that it does not have to be that complicated. There's no need for you to spend another day beating yourself up or thinking that you are a failure. You can do this! I am proof! I will walk with you through this process to help you achieve the lasting success you desire. You might even find that losing weight can be fun!

> Creating lasting change in any area of life can be challenging, but the good news is that it does not have to be that complicated.

This book is just for you. My story and the things that I have learned over the years will serve as a guide to help you discover your personalized "formula" to lose weight and keep it off. You will discover some secret ingredients that will empower you, so that you will make the process of losing weight less complicated and more enjoyable.

Throughout this book, you will find questions and activities that will help you on your adventure. This book is meant to be your source of encouragement, a go-to-reference guide, and a life-long resource you can use at any stage of your process. I recommend reading through the entire book before you work through the activities. Then, go back through the book, starting with the sections you feel you need the most, depending on where you are in the process. Choose one activity to work on at a time. Once you've worked on that activity for a few days, you might start adding others one at a time.

This isn't meant to be a program that makes you feel overwhelmed or restricted. Some of the activities will work for you and others will not. This is okay. I want you to discover what works for you! You will add one piece of progress onto another until you see the results you want.

Get some friends together, encourage each other and discuss some of the sections of the book. Be sure to come visit me at facebook.com/marylouhelps for daily inspiration and to join a community with like-minded individuals!

1

Find Your Own "Why"

A strategy that helped me tremendously in losing weight was to find my "why." It had to be something "bigger" than achieving a smaller number on the scale. Losing weight was simply the benefit that came from working on my "why."

> *Don't try to keep yourself motivated by something that "should" motivate you.*

Discovering your "why" is essential. It's your "why" that will keep you moving forward on those tough days. Don't try to keep yourself motivated by something that "should" motivate you.

For instance, if you're saying something like, "I should be motivated by ____ or I should be doing ____!", then you're probably choosing a "why" that won't work for you. There isn't a right or wrong "why." Your "why" is what will motivate you for the long term.

 # Activity 1.0

Think of all of the benefits that can be achieved through the process of losing weight.

1. What is one or more benefit that people could experience when they lose weight?

I encourage you today... dream BIG!! List whatever comes to mind. Remember, you are trying to find what motivates YOU, so don't worry about your answer being right or wrong.

FIRST, check off any of the benefits below that you feel apply to you.

- ☐ More energy
- ☐ Ability to keep up with younger people
- ☐ Feeling more comfortable in clothes that fit me well
- ☐ Ability to fit in smaller seats
- ☐ Ability to finish something that I start
- ☐ Spiritual or personal growth
- ☐ Ability to walk around people who are sitting without asking them to move
- ☐ Pants or legs don't rub together when I walk
- ☐ Feeling better about myself
- ☐ Feeling at peace with what I value
- ☐ Food not being my first choice to fill needs
- ☐ Making a difference in the lives of others
- ☐ Setting an example for family, friends, etc.
- ☐ Able to handle stress better
- ☐ Able to serve God more with more energy

☐ Growing stronger during stressful times

☐ Able to more easily delay gratification

☐ Not worrying about family and friends being concerned about my physical or emotional health

☐ Having mental energy for other things than weight, food, etc.

SECOND, add to this list anything that comes to mind.

THIRD, review what you circled and pick one or two that are the most appealing to you right now. Write them down.

FOURTH, look at what you just chose and list some additional benefits that they could provide.

For example, if your choice was that your friends or family would be less concerned about your physical or emotional health, one additional benefit would be that you would be able to lift the burden of that concern from them.

Many times the first thing that comes to mind isn't what is truly motivating you. So, you might want to consider continuing to further identify the "benefits of the benefits of the benefits." Don't get stuck overanalyzing this. The goal is to find what motivates you RIGHT NOW and then revisit this regularly.

These types of goals and motivations are more likely than other types to give you the desire to persevere. When weight loss is the goal, there can be an emphasis on what we don't like about ourselves, and that never brings lasting change. Make sure that your "why" is something positive and will provide benefits to you.

The following steps will be helpful:

1. Write down how these would benefit you.

2. Identify what it will cost you if you did not have these benefits.

3. Take a moment to think through the questions that you just answered. Write down what is motivating to you right now.

That's it! Your "why" is whatever is motivating you right now. It's important that you **remind yourself of your "why" regularly**, so be sure to come back to this exercise. You may even want to post a visual of your "why" so you will be reminded of it often. Expect God to meet you right where you are, and He will empower you.

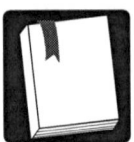

Think about what this verse means to you today.
Write it down, make a list or sketch it out.
"No eye has seen, no ear has heard, and no mind has imagined what God has prepared for those who love him."
1 Corinthians 2:9 (NLT)

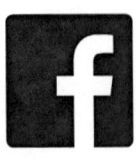

Let's Connect: I would love to know what your "why" is. Remember that there is no such thing as a perfect answer. It's simply what is motivating you right now! Stop in at facebook.com/marylouhelps and share what's motivating you right now!

2

One Size Does NOT Fit All

Have you ever felt frustrated when others are losing weight, but the process they are using doesn't work for you? Did you feel that YOU were the problem? Perhaps you even flooded yourself with a host of negative messages. It is so easy to turn the blame back on ourselves when we don't get the results we want. What works for them may not be what works best for you!

> *Almost any program or book can offer something that is beneficial to one person, but can actually "backfire" for another person.*

Instead of getting frustrated with yourself, seek the solutions that will fit your individual needs.

I remember feeling that I was the problem when I tried to lose weight and later tried to keep it off. I finally realized that I was just trying to do what worked for someone else, and what they were doing was simply not a fit for me at the time. I discovered that instead of strictly following a particular program, I could make tweaks so that it would work for me.

This reality was freeing for me and helped me to have great results.

Almost any program or book can offer something that is beneficial to one person, but can actually "backfire" for another person.

 ## Activity 2.1

FIRST, take a minute and picture yourself in the future. You have lost weight, and you have kept it off. You think back to how you lost the weight, and _____ was NOT on YOUR list of strategies that you used, yet you still had success.

What things come to mind to fill in the blank? To give examples, here are some things that could be on your list:

- Exercise/treadmill
- Cooking/extra time it takes to cook
- Weighing and measuring food
- Counting calories
- Avoiding a specific food
- Eating every 3 hours
- Keeping a food journal
- Denying yourself simple pleasures like going out to eat

SECOND, write down some more things to add to this list, whatever it is that comes to mind.

THIRD, circle your favorites.

FOURTH, narrow it down to ONE choice, one strategy that you did not have to do, yet you still got there! Write it down.

You might find that you don't ever have to use the strategy that you most dread. For now, simply try other things. As you work through this book, I encourage you to:

1. Pray and ask God to show you one thing that would make a difference for you right now.

2. Avoid overanalyzing it. Just start where you are willing.

3. Try not to be overwhelmed by thinking that your journey would require you to copy my journey or anyone else's. Making ONE change is powerful.

Think about what this verse means to you today.
Write it down, make a list or sketch it out.
"For we are God's masterpiece. He has created us anew in Christ Jesus, so we can do the good things he planned for us long ago." **Ephesians 2:10 (NLT)**

Write what this quote means to you today.

"Everybody is a Genius. But if you judge a fish by its ability to climb a tree, it will live its whole life believing it is stupid"
– **Albert Einstein.**

Activity 2.2

What you can say to someone who gives you advice or possible solutions? Write it down.

For example:

- "I've been there done that…"
- "Thank you for your input."
- "Thanks, but as with so many things, I need to find my own way."
- "There is so much information these days with weight loss. I am finding my way and appreciate your input. I will consider your suggestion. Thank you."
- "Thank you for sharing what has helped you. I will give it some thought."
- "Maybe I will consider that, however, I am sticking to my current plan to see how well it works."

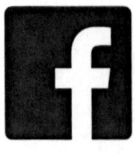 ***Let's Connect:*** Stop in at <u>facebook.com/marylouhelps</u> and share one change that you are making today.

3

Adventure Buddies

"Two people are better off than one, for they can help each other succeed. If one person falls, the other can reach out and help. But someone who falls alone is in real trouble," **Ecclesiastes 4:9-12 (NLT)**

It's essential to have a healthy connection with at least one other person about your weight loss journey. This must be someone who will not try to fix you, someone who believes in you, who accepts you unconditionally, and will speak the truth to you with grace. This connection could be established through a community of like-minded people. Your community might include joining a group that is already formed, forming your own group, or having one Adventure Buddy. Any of these are helpful.

> *It's essential to have a healthy connection with at least one other person about your weight loss journey.*

"We know from research that growth is actually contagious so if you want to reach your goals, you've got to get around people that are going in the same direction you want to be going and you will catch the success. The data proves it."

"The biggest mistake people make is trying to accomplish the goal based on commitment and trying harder. That will fail.

Instead, get together with people who are already accomplishing what you want to accomplish. If you want to become healthy, you have to surround yourself with a group of people that are getting healthy and you have to be connected to a community that is doing what you want to do." [1]

– Dr. Henry Cloud

Questions to ask each other:

1. What comes to your mind when you hear the word "accountability?"

2. What doesn't work well for you (such as being given a pat answer, being judged based on your food choices, being asked what you ate, being asked what you weigh, etc.)?

3. What works well for you (such as someone being direct, not being rushed for an answer, etc.)?

4. How do you want to connect with each other between your regularly scheduled times?

Keep the lines of communication open so that you can be real with each other along the way. The best way for someone to "learn" from you is for you to share what you are working on right now. Refrain from giving advice or tips to someone else.

Remember:
- We each have our own journey in life that brought us to this point. What works for someone else, might not work for you.
- Resist comparing yourself or your results to anyone else.
- Be honest and real.

- Daily put positive things into your mind.
- Make an action step every day.
- Learn about yourself and what works for you in the process.
- Let go of what doesn't work for you.
- If you want to have someone else follow-up with you regarding the choices you are making, do it in a way that empowers you.
- Have a friend or professional that you trust ask you questions that you want them to ask and be ready to be truthful with them.

If you want to have a group that does not use a scale, then be sure to remind people ahead of time that the purpose of this group is not to weigh in, to talk about how much you weigh, or to talk about how much you may or may not have lost. Many times people don't realize how they can make someone else feel based on how they talk about their own weight. Someone can make a facial expression, use a certain tone of voice or words to put themselves down based on their weight, and they may not realize how it can make someone feel, if that other person weighs more than they do.

If the scale is empowering to anyone in the group, encourage them to have someone else outside of the group celebrate their results on the scale. If your community decides to use a scale or talk about the numbers on the scale, please make that allow that time to be optional, and schedule it at the beginning or end of the session when people can come later or leave early.

Discuss:
If your community is talking about the food itself, i.e. what foods are being eaten:

- Realistically look at the time that is spent. How much of it is talking about food such as what to eat, what not to eat, how to fix it, when to eat it, etc?

- Does the conversation leave you feeling empowered to do what works for you, or are you leaving more enamored with food or even more confused than before?
- How much time do you talk about things other than food?

Talk about more than just the food. For example:

- Take notice about what you are thinking when you make the food choice and talk about that
- Talk about what you are learning about yourself and what works for you
- Share if you are feeling deprived or defeated. If so, come up with one strategy you can do today to change that

Think about what this verse means to you today.
Write it down, make a list or sketch it out.
"The Lord will guide you continually, giving you water when you are dry and restoring your strength. You will be like a well-watered garden, like an ever-flowing spring." **Isaiah 58:11 (NLT)**

For the Adventure Buddy:

You might not be struggling with weight issues yourself, but you care about someone who does have this struggle. If that is the case, the most important thing you have to offer is respect and unconditional love.

 **Activity 3.1**

Ask each other, "What is one specific example of how I can show you respect and unconditional love?"

 **Activity 3.2**

You are out to eat with someone who says they want to lose weight and you don't think they have made a good selection for their food choice. What do you do? Write it down and discuss it with someone else.

Tip: If you are a buddy or part of a support team to someone, say something like, "I would love to learn how to talk about this sensitive issue, would you be willing to teach me? Could we start with you sharing one thing that I could say differently?" The person might not respond right away, it can take time. Just continue to be available without being pushy.

One way to show respect is to remove the words "Can" or "Can't" when it comes to talking about food.

For example, if you say any of the following:

"Can you eat that?"

"What foods can you not have on your diet?"

Replace that with asking questions like:

"What food changes are you making?"

"What is one new choice are you going to make this week when it comes to food?"

These types of questions are more empowering because the focus is on the choices the person is making rather than on the food itself being a "good" or "bad" choice.

Ask yourself these questions regularly:

- Do I nag someone about their health, size or eating habits?
- Do I feel that I have to take control, because no one seems to be doing anything about the situation?
- Do I tell someone something they should be doing or should be eating?
- Do I feel helpless in offering assistance, so I do nothing?

- Do I judge someone based on their size and come to a conclusion? For example do I assume they don't care, or don't work hard enough?
- Do I feel that I know the only solution that should work for everyone?
- Do I feel rejected if I have prepared food and someone does not want to eat it?

4

Set Goals That Work For You

Have you found it helpful to set goals on how much weight you are going to lose? What about setting a goal about how long it will take? Does a weekly weigh-in work well for you?

Some people do well setting goals based on their goal weight and how long it will take. Some also do well with a weekly weigh-in. If you find that works well, keep it up – good for you!

I didn't weigh myself or set weight loss goals until I was involved in programs that encouraged or required those steps. I wasn't sure what goals to set or how long it would take to reach them, so I just followed the plans.

It was very frustrating to me when my results didn't fit into what I felt "should" have worked for me. I would either quit or I would tolerate the feeling of frustration and assume that things had to be that way in order for me to lose weight.

I remember walking into the room and there would be a line of people getting ready to be weighed. I felt as if we were cattle being lined up. It just didn't feel human to me. I wanted results, so I continued assuming this is how it had to be.

If I felt the results were positive, I was encouraged. If they were a fraction less than what I had hoped for, I would easily become frustrated or discouraged.

To try to "fix" my frustration, I would:
- Try harder
- Either exercise more, eat less, or both
- Ignore hunger
- Add more rules to my plan

I continued to attend the meetings because I liked being around other people who were on the same journey as I was and I could learn tips that could make a difference for me. Yet, it really frustrated me when people cheered about their results on the scale and how long it took them to achieve these results. I can remember many times hearing people cheering about their weight loss numbers and then hear the whispers of how they "cheated that week."

I became even more focused on my weight loss numbers and tried to figure out how quickly I should be able to lose weight. I felt that the problem must have been me. I must not be "normal." It was a terrible place to be mentally, believing that I was always the problem but also not knowing how to get the results that I desired.

Eventually, I had to give up the scale for 3 months as a result of foot surgery, because I could not stand on the scale. I was still able to lose weight, however, even while recovering from the surgery.

Using a scale is not necessary for everyone. I am able to work with more people as a result of that insight. Scale or no scale, it really doesn't matter. What matters is what works for each individual!

If using the scale works for you, but you want to tweak the weekly weigh-in, here are some options for you:
- You don't have to find out what you weigh each time. You can close your eyes, turn around or just ask to not see the numbers
- You can weigh and/or measure yourself at home once a month

- You may choose not to set goals based on how long it takes
- You can celebrate whatever result that you get, rather than require specific results in order to be satisfied
- You can celebrate that you have an opportunity to learn about yourself and what can work for you
- You can chose groups that minimize the cheering about results on the scale

> ... look at the results as a gift. If they happen to be quick results, that's just a nice bonus, but it is NOT a requirement.

It can be empowering to look at the results as a gift. If they happen to be quick results, that's just a nice bonus, but it is NOT a requirement. I discovered that it was better for me to set goals on the things I could control (my actions, choices, and responses), rather than setting goals on what I had no control over (losing a certain amount of weight each week).

 **Activity 4.1**

What will you do when there is no longer the "reward" of a smaller number on the scale or a smaller clothing size once the goal is achieved? Write it down, talk to someone about it.

 **Activity 4.2**

Try any of these and write down your thoughts:
- Embrace what works for you. If setting goals based on the amount of weight you will lose in a specific amount of time works for you, then go for it.
- Accept that it's a myth that hard work equals radical results.
- Realize that you don't have complete control over how fast the scale changes.
- Make plans for what you will do when you get discouraged.

Set goals based on what you truly have control over such as your actions, choices, and responses.

For example:
- What are you doing to proactively change what you think while you lose the weight?

- What are you doing to be more active than you were last week?
- What change are you making in your food choices?
- What are you doing to change how you respond to stressful situations?

 **Activity 4.3**

Write down a goal that you are going to pursue this week.

 **Think about what this verse means to you today.** Write it down, make a list or sketch it out.

"Trust in the Lord with all your heart; do not depend on your own understanding. Seek his will in all you do, and he will show you which path to take." **Proverbs 3:5-6 (NLT)**

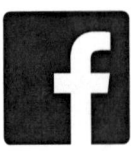 ***Let's Connect:*** Stop in at facebook.com/marylouhelps and share a goal that can be set based on something that is truly within your control.

5

Empower or Backfire

When I followed programs that counted calories or gave food a numerical value, I found that losing weight became a math problem. I focused too much on doing the math and found that I was missing out on many of the other tools I could have been using. Since counting calories backfired for me, I eventually stopped counting them.

The process of focusing on the numbers caused me to:

- Think about food more than I ever had in my life
- Not eat some foods that were good for me just because they were higher in calories
- Focus on volume too much. Volume became too important
- Miss out the power of smaller portions that tasted great and were very satisfying
- Miss out on really savoring food and simply enjoying it
- Ignore being satisfied and fail to stop eating when I was satisfied. In other words, I was eating too much
- Ignore Hunger. When I was truly hungry, I did not eat, just so I could lose weight

What I learned about myself:

- My old way of craving food made me eat past my level of satisfaction
- I no longer need volume in order to be satisfied

- Feeling that I had to eat when I was not hungry encouraged me to turn off my hunger cues
- I didn't have to eat just to make sure that I wouldn't be hungry later

What about food plans, programs or products? Any of these can be very effective if they are looked at as a tool to help you, rather than the one and only solution. Remember, you are unique and your weight-loss adventure will be what works for you. You may have tried one of the many food plans on the market. The question you should ask is, "Do food plans work for me?"

You might do very well with a specific food plan, following it exactly, or tweaking it. Please do not over-analyze this. If you are already using a food plan that is working well for you, stick with it and consider adding one of the other tools in the book to make your plan even more effective for you.

> *I was actually training my mind to think compulsively about many things in life, not just food.*

It's important to do what works for your personality and your lifestyle. If you are a free spirit and you try to do what works for someone who loves high structure, it's not going to fit you well. You will be left feeling frustrated and defeated.

Food really wasn't on my mind before I starting dieting. When I tried a "diet" or a "food plan," I simply listened to what I was "told" to eat rather than taking personal ownership for my food choices. Food preoccupied my mind more than it ever had before.

At the time, I did not realize that something very unhealthy was happening to me. I was actually training my mind to think compulsively about many things in life, not just food. The compulsive thinking caused problems for me in other areas of my life that were unrelated to my weight.

Food plans are not necessarily bad. They work well for many people and I learned how to tweak food plans when I used them. I also learned how to eat intuitively which requires no food plans whatsoever. Listening to your body and what it needs is a powerful weight loss tool. It may take some practice but the result is very freeing and satisfying.

 **Activity 5.0**

Do you feel that you can trust yourself with your food choices? If not, what would it be like if you did? Do you ever feel that a food plan restricts you and makes you feel as if you have to have permission to eat certain foods or not? If so, what can you do today to change that thought? Write your answers.

Think about what this verse means to you today.
Write it down, make a list or sketch it out.
"But those who trust in the Lord will find new strength. They will soar high on wings like eagles. They will run and not grow weary. They will walk and not faint." **Isaiah 40:31 (NLT)**

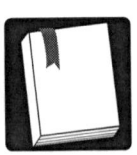

Think about what this verse means to you today. Write it down, make a list or sketch it out.
"The thief's purpose is to steal and kill and destroy. My purpose is to give them a rich and satisfying life." **John 10:10 (NLT)**

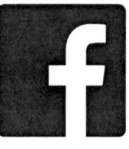 ***Let's Connect:*** Stop in at <u>facebook.com/marylouhelps</u> and share one weight loss strategy that works for someone else, but you don't like to use it yourself.

6

I'm Stressed! Who Has the Chocolate?

Have you ever thought, "I'm having a bad day, I deserve something delicious?" Maybe you were bored and found yourself looking for food? Stress can certainly trigger food cravings. Has food ever temporarily calmed stress for you? Maybe it temporarily helped you to feel a little less bored, angry, lonely, or tired?

> *The more that I turned to food under stress, the weaker I became and the less stress that I could handle.*

Food can be very calming and a "quick fix" when you are feeling stressed. You feel better, even if it is just temporary. I used to use food as source of stress relief. The more that I turned to food under stress, the weaker I became and the less stress that I could handle.

You can also make some choices to become a stronger person even during stress. Be prepared for the next time you are faced with something that you find stressful by practicing one of these statements before the stress comes.

 **Activity 6.1**

Think to yourself or say out loud, "Thank you for this opportunity to...":

- practice saying no
- set an example for my children that food isn't a good source of stress relief
- grow stronger
- develop my character
- make it easier for me to say no next time
- change my cravings

> *Each time you do this, you make great progress towards not using food as a source of stress relief.*

If you want it to be short and sweet, just a simple "Thank you" will do!

Each time you do this, you make great progress towards not using food as a source of stress relief. You will find that you are reprogramming your mind to think positive, proactive thoughts. It doesn't mean that you will necessarily be grateful for the specific stressful situation, but the circumstance will no longer fuel your craving for more food.

 **Activity 6.2**

What about other emotions? Maybe you are bored, or you've had a disappointment, or you are lonely, angry or tired. What could you do then? Write down something that you can do when you are feeling any of these emotions.

One option would be to feel the emotion, even if it's just for a minute. We can't selectively numb emotions. If you numb the bad stuff such as grief, fear or disappointment, you also numb joy, gratitude and happiness. [2]

 **Think about what this verse means to you today.**
Write it down, make a list or sketch it out.
"Fix your thoughts on what is true, and honorable, and right, and pure, and lovely, and admirable. Think about things that are excellent and worthy of praise."
Philippians 4:8

Trigger Foods and Stress Relief

Food can still change my mood. However, it's not very often that I use it to change how I am feeling. One of the things that helped me in the beginning was to be honest with myself about the types of foods that I turned to when I was under stress.

I realized that I already had more than my share of those foods and it wouldn't hurt me to temporarily wait to eat them while I learned some new skills. That was helpful for me. Others find that they do fine with occasionally having their trigger foods. It's important to be real with yourself and do what works for you.

Eventually, I came to a place in my life where I could tell when certain foods would trigger stronger food cravings. I also could recognize when I would be able to handle the trigger foods without it causing me to have an uncontrollable appetite.

One day, we were having a celebration, and I knew that I would do fine enjoying a "trigger" food. Just as the food was about to be served, I received some very, stressful and upsetting news. I knew that I could still have the food if I wanted to, yet I knew that I wouldn't really enjoy it since I was so stressed. If I had it, I would regret that decision later. Having the food would have fueled my desire for more food later and would have made me feel even more stressed. I was very glad that I chose to wait. I really enjoyed the food later.

Have you ever felt that cravings for food were something that you had to harness, control or fix?

Cravings

Have you ever felt that cravings for food were something that you had to harness, control or fix? What you crave in food can actually help you identify what you really need. God is "wooing you" to a gift that He wants to give you in the moment.

 **Activity 6.3**

When a craving comes, pray, "God, what is it that I need right now? What is it that you have for me that you want to give me?"

 **Activity 6.4**

To change your cravings for food, start replacing "self-denial" with an acceptance of what you need at that moment. Make a list of things that you can do that don't include food.

Here are some examples: call someone, go for a walk, rest, read, clean, listen to music, take a 5 minute break, etc.

The next time you are craving food, do one of the activities on your list.

Write down what you get from the activity.

For example: I felt joy, I felt nurtured, I felt comfort.

Celebrate that you filled yourself with what you needed at the moment!

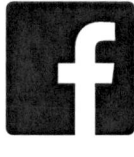 ***Let's Connect:*** Stop in at facebook.com/marylouhelps and share your ideas for what you can do to fill a craving that doesn't include food.

 # Activity 6.5

Try this experiment to see what it does for your intensity or frequency of food cravings:

Choose ONE of these to intentionally work on this week. Put today's date by the one you choose.

_____ Drink more water.

_____ Pay attention to what foods keep you satisfied longer and which ones don't.

_____ Brush your teeth when feeling tempted to snack. It will change the taste in your mouth and decrease the desire to eat something.

_____ Notice if certain foods increase hunger when you eat them certain times of day.

_____ Notice if your food cravings are reduced by exercise or moving around any particular time of the day.

_____ Notice if a more natural form of the same food is more satisfying.

_____ Purposely slow down when eating.

_____ Set your fork or spoon down between bites.

_____ Notice if certain food combinations increase or decrease how long you are satisfied.

Optional add-on: When you eat something write down what it is or take a picture. Mark down the time of day.

 **Think about what this verse means to you today.**
Write it down, make a list or sketch it out.
"He gives power to the weak and strength to the powerless."
Isaiah 40:29 (NLT)

What are You Really Getting From Food?

There are so many enjoyable things about food:

- Texture
- Appearance
- Special memory associated with that food
- Smell
- Physical boost, even if short-lived
- Taste

Simply enjoy what you like about the food and keep the decision to eat it separate from what you enjoy about it.

Some experts say that creamy foods can mean you need nurturing, while craving crunchy foods shows a need for some positive aggression.

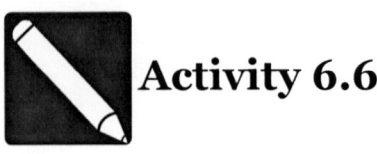 **Activity 6.6**

For one day, notice things that you enjoy about the food itself and write down anything that you notice.

 **Activity 6.7**

Try this experiment for a few days:

FIRST, notice how you feel after you eat when you aren't really sure if you are hungry or not. You might feel comforted, or loved, or you might be able to release some aggression. Write down what food you ate and what you received from eating it.

SECOND, add ONE of these and make your own:

A. "God, I recognize that I want fun right now, this _____ would be fun, please show me something else that would be fun instead." You can do the same with nurturing and comfort, etc.

B. A simple thought: fun is good (comfort is good). Do I really want to get fun or comfort from this food right now?

C. What other food could be fun or comforting right now? For example: An apple can provide a crunch or sweetness.

Making Your Food Work FOR You

Changing my food choices helped with my cravings. I learned which foods increased my cravings and which ones made me feel more satisfied after eating them. My taste buds and cravings changed as I changed the types of food that I ate.

Some things I learned along the way:
- I know what foods and what time of day certain foods work for me.
- I can recognize what portions work for me without ignoring hunger.
- As I recognize how much food will typically satisfy me, I realize that each day could be a little different. Some days I am hungrier than I am other days, and I don't avoid eating for concern of gaining weight.
- It's not about following a set of rules. It's an adventure.

# Activity 6.8

Watch for one opportunity today to give yourself what you want, need or desire. Then follow through, even if it's for a few seconds and see what happens to your cravings.

7

Food is No Longer Center Stage

In the past, I thought about food a lot. Now, it no longer "calls my name." I can go anywhere and I rarely notice the food that is there. I would have never imagined that my life would be filled with this freedom. You can enjoy the same freedom, too!

National speaker, author and executive coach Dwight Bain had an exciting opportunity to apply for a one-year speaking contract. The company brought about 12 speakers in for an event and listened to their speaking abilities. Dwight assumed they would make their decision based on the quality of the applicants' public speaking.

The speakers were taken to a fancy restaurant and told they could eat whatever they wanted. The company watched how the speakers ate. Were they filling up the plate to overflow or were they talking to the executives about what they wanted to accomplish with their company?

He and most of the other speakers were more interested in food and just chatting with everyone else. The only exception was one guy who was paying attention. He wasn't there for the food, he was there to talk about the company.

Dwight asked him how he got the contract since he wasn't the best speaker. He said it was because he did not focus on the food, but, instead, he talked to them about their company. He figured that he could buy his dinner later. [3]

I could really relate to this story. In the past, I would have been just like the other speakers, really focusing on the food. Now, my response would be more like the guy who ended up getting the contract. I would take personal responsibility for what I was going to eat.

> *Food just isn't as big of a deal now.*

I would be very focused on enjoying the people there. If I ate the food, I would really be enjoying it, but not likely as much as I would enjoy the company. I am likely to forget to get extra food, and I might even forget to eat everything that I ordered. Instead, I could eat before I go or just eat something after, or I could ask the waiter if I can order at the end and get it to go. I know that I am responsible for my own nourishment needs. Food just isn't as big of a deal now. Enjoying people is much more important to me.

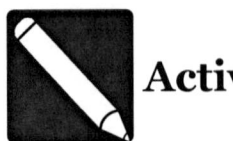 ## Activity 7.1

What is one thing that you will do today that will remind you to enjoy things other than just the food in a social setting? Write your answer.

 **Think about what this verse means to you today.**
Write it down, make a list or sketch it out.
"Where the Spirit of the Lord is, there is freedom."
2 Corinthians 3:17 (NIV)

Reboot Your Thinking

Part of lasting weight loss success involves examining the messages you listen to while losing weight. Focus on the power of your choices rather than on the food itself.

> *The process takes just split seconds and it's very easy to do.*

You have probably had problems with an electronic device and found that something as simple as turning it off, unplugging it, and then plugging it back in, makes the device work much better. We can do the same with the way we think about the process of losing weight. You can take a thought that you have, make a slight change to it, and it can consequently reboot the way that you think. I have found this to be a very powerful tool. The process takes just split seconds and it's very easy to do.

I remember being around food, being tempted and resisting many times by telling myself, "I can't have that. It's not on my diet." I might have had temporary success by resisting, yet I felt deprived, which caused more problems.

I rebooted my thinking by changing that thought to, "I can have it if I want it. If I say no this time, though, it will be easier next time."

It did not take long before it became easier, even to the point that I barely noticed food. The pull and the temptation were greatly reduced by making this simple change.

Some important things that help me when I use this technique:

- When I thought, "I can have it if I want it," I had to believe it.
- My phrase was the opposite of what didn't work for me, "I can't have that, it's not on my diet."
- Saying that it wasn't on my diet and that I couldn't have it made me feel deprived. I also felt that the food itself was more powerful than my right to have it. This made the food even more appealing and made me less empowered.
- I added, "it will be easier next time" because that was very important to me. I was tired of the cravings. I was tired of looking for the food. I really wanted that to change.
- I practiced saying my phrase out loud when I was not facing a food choice and it started coming to me quickly when I needed it. What we believe more than anything is what we hear ourselves say, so saying that out loud helped me to believe it.

# Activity 7.2

What about you? Do you notice what it is that you are saying to yourself when you are in the midst of a food temptation? Write it down or speak it into the voice recorder on your phone so you can remember it and change it. If you don't know what it is, then pay attention the next few times until you remember what it is that you are thinking.

Now, change it into something more empowering. Don't overanalyze trying to get the perfect phrase; it just needs to feel positive to you when you hear yourself say it. Tweak what you are saying now.

Here are some examples:

- Change "I will start tomorrow" or "why bother" or "this one time doesn't really matter" to: "This choice matters!"
- Change "I will end up quitting" to: "I am more than a conqueror!"
- Change "Just this one more time" to: "Do I want to be more empowered, deprived or defeated?"
- Change "I'm stressed, that looks delicious" to "Thank you for the opportunity to grow stronger."
- Change "I want it NOW!" to "I am choosing to practice waiting, it will get easier."
- Change "This is too hard" to "I can do all things through Christ who gives me strength."

Make your own phrase. If you aren't sure what to do, ask someone to help you. Start practicing your phrase when you do not have food in front of you. Then practice and keep practicing. It will be worth it. Rebooting your thinking just in one thought will start the ball rolling, and before you know it food will not call your name as loudly.

 **Activity 7.3**

When a craving is strong, try this tip from a Family Talk Interview with Allison Bottke.

> Stop and say to God, "I know that I shouldn't eat it, but I want it." Ask Him to show you what you can do now. You may be thinking, "I feel awful, I am very lonely, but I want that burger." Ask God to help you fill your thoughts with His Word. If you are driving, you may even need to pull the car over and ask God for additional help. Wait for ten minutes. Tell yourself that if you have to have the burger in 10 minutes, then you'll get it. When the ten minutes are up, choose to wait another ten minutes. You'll quickly begin to realize that you have more control than you thought. [4]

Think about what this verse means to you today.
Write it down, make a list or sketch it out.
"For I can do everything through Christ, who gives me strength." **Philippians 4:13(NLT)**

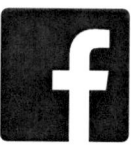

Let's Connect: Stop in at <u>facebook.com/marylouhelps</u> and share what new words or phrase you are using to reboot your thinking.

8

A New and Easier Relationship with Food

When I was a child, a healthy relationship with food was modeled in our home. Just to name a few things:
- We had wholesome foods at home.
- No foods were off limits or bad.
- Food was not used as a reward or punishment.
- I don't ever remember anyone being on a diet.
- There were not messages of depriving self in order to lose weight.
- I didn't see any emotional eating.
- My parents had plenty of ways to show love, security or comfort that did not include food.
- We had celebrations that included food. The food itself was just not the center of attention.

As a child, I was the only overweight person in my family. I might have eaten a little differently than the rest of my family, but if I did, I had no idea that I was doing that. I don't remember anything significant about my eating habits as a child. I may have overeaten, or I may have been an emotional eater, but I wasn't aware of it then.

> "Both adults and children eat in response to happy and uncomfortable feelings. It is a learned behavior that we either model from others or discover on our own. We hurt, we eat,

and then feel better, or we are happy and eat to celebrate. The cycle is repeated. Once emotional eating becomes habitual, we overeat without thinking or understanding why we put food in our mouths." [5] – Dr. Linda Mintle

I really didn't think much about food or my weight until my mid 20's when I gained a lot of weight and then started working on losing it. Twenty years of yo-yo dieting changed my thought process about food, which led me to having a very unhealthy relationship with food. Now, I really enjoy food again and more importantly, I enjoy living at peace with food.

Think about what this verse means to you today.
Write it down, make a list or sketch it out.
"There is no condemnation for those who belong to Christ Jesus." **Romans 8:1 (NLT)**

Feeling Deprived

I used to feel that I had to make myself hungry in order to lose weight. I remember being very cranky when I was hungry. I felt very deprived. When you are on a "diet", do you feel that you have to deprive yourself? If so, has that worked for you?

> ... denying myself food made me unable to hear God wooing me to something good that He had for me in the moment.

When we change our eating habits, it does take a bit of sacrifice in the moment to give up what you are craving and turn to what you truly want, need or desire. When I quickly turned to food, it made it harder to know what I truly wanted. In the past, denying myself food made me unable to hear God wooing me to something good that He had for me in the moment. There were small, subtle shifts that happened over time and I didn't realize what was happening.

I had stopped listening to my needs and honoring what I truly needed in the moment. I would eat because I thought I was hungry. Food offered a temporary fix, but left me feeling empty afterward. This then led me to distrust myself and ultimately caused me to not hear what God desired to give me in each moment. Denying myself food when I was truly hungry also led to me denying myself other legitimate needs, such as rest, relaxation, and fun.

Once I started replacing "self-denial" and filling myself with the good things that I needed at the moment, I made great progress in redirecting my craving for food. Have you ever felt that you had to miss out on all of the joys of eating just to lose weight?

> "We should be able to enjoy a beautiful ice cream sundae. Eating it is not wrong or bad. It is okay to enjoy the moment the spoon hits your mouth and you taste the flavors. But we don't want to act impulsively and eat things we really don't want or need – especially if we're going to regret it later." [6]
> – Dr. Linda Mintle

 ## Activity 8.1

It's important to really enjoy eating. It's possible to lose weight and still really enjoy your food. Brainstorm with others and list as many things that you can think of that you enjoy about eating. Let's see how many things we can come up with as an online community.

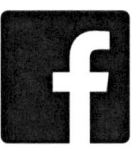 *Let's Connect:* Stop in at facebook.com/marylouhelps and share one thing that you enjoy about eating.

Is This "Hunger" Really for Food?

Sometimes it is difficult to identity if you are hungry for food or if you are eating for a different reason. When I wanted to lose weight, I thought that I had to just ignore hunger and live with it. That didn't work well for me in the long run. When I wasn't trying to lose weight, I didn't pay attention to hunger and just ate impulsively. That didn't work well for me either.

Here's a simple strategy that helped me:

- I would simply make myself pause, just for a split second and ask myself, "Could I be hungry, angry, lonely, tired or bored?"
- At first, I really didn't know which one I was feeling. I just started noticing that I could be feeling something different than hunger at the time.
- Just taking the split second before deciding to eat or not was very powerful to me.
- After a while, I started to recognize, "Oh, I'm bored," or "I am angry," etc.
- I would have a variety of simple strategies ready to use in the moment. You can use the list that you made in Activity 6.4.

> *The more I did this, the more food lost its power over me.*

Those split seconds it took to pause before eating was very powerful for me. Over time, I started to recognize things that were more fulfilling than food in that particular moment. The more I did this, the more food lost its power over me.

Eat When Hungry, Stop When Satisfied

A great strategy to add to any weight loss solution is to eat when you are hungry, and stop when you are satisfied. This sounds like it should be so simple, but many times we have lost the ability to recognize the signals.

Here are some tips that can be helpful:

- Losing weight can be an adventure. Learn as you go.
- Don't be hard on yourself or expect perfection.
- Don't add a new "rule" such as eating "only" when hungry and stopping when satisfied.

This is an important skill to learn, but it does take some time. I still occasionally overeat, and don't always quickly recognize when I have gone past feeling satisfied. I am not legalistic about it. If I overeat, I learn from it. I tell myself, "That much food made me too full last time so next time I slow down and recognize when I'm satisfied."

Losing weight can be an adventure.

 **Activity 8.2**

Try this activity. It's not meal time and you start thinking about food, quickly ask yourself any ONE of these questions:

- Is this a habit, does it look good, or am I just used to buying a snack at a check-out counter?
- What do I need? A quick break or a smaller amount of food can work.

- Do I want to feel more empowered or more deprived, defeated or discouraged?
- The food smells good, so enjoy the smell. The decision to eat it or not is not attached to how good it smells.
- The food is pretty. Enjoy the way that it looks. Your decision to eat it or not is not attached to the look of the food.
- Someone else wants you to eat. Tell yourself, "I have a choice right now. I can do what's best for me."
- Look away from the food while making a decision. Quickly turn your attention somewhere else. Then make your decision.
- Ask yourself, "Am I eating this impulsively or do I really want to eat this?"

"Eating impulsively can add unwanted pounds and bring guilt. Enjoying the moment doesn't mean losing control over your brain." [7] – Dr. Linda Mintle

What about eating when you are not hungry to prevent being hungry later? Do what works well for you. If you know that keeping food available or eating every 3 hours helps you to not go overboard later, then stick with that.

Some things to think about:
- It doesn't take a lot of food to curb extreme hunger later.
- Notice what foods or food combinations tend to keep you more satisfied.
- What do you do when the foods that fuel you aren't available? Do you panic and fear becoming too hungry later?

Even though eating before getting hungry can work well for some people, you might not be one of those people and that's OK. Do what works for you. Sometimes, making yourself eat when you are not hungry could cause you to think about food even more, or make your hunger cues more difficult to notice. What does being hungry or feeling satisfied really feel like?

 **Activity 8.3**

1. Write down the options you have when you get hungry.

2. Pick one of these numbers on "The Hunger Scale" (see next page) and watch for feeling that way this week. Notice what it really feels like and write it down.

Tip: I don't recommend that you start with numbers 5 or 6. They can be the hardest to recognize. Feeling satisfied doesn't feel all that much different than mildly hungry.

The Hunger Scale

1	Starving, dizzy, irritable
2	Very hungry, unable to concentrate
3	Hungry, ready to eat
4	Beginning signals of hunger
5	Comfortable, neither hungry nor full
6	Comfortably full, satisfied
7	Very full, feels like you have overeaten
8	Uncomfortably full, feel stuffed
9	Very full, very uncomfortable, need to loosen your clothes
10	Stuffed to the point of feeling sick

As I've learned to listen to my hunger cues, I stopped making myself hungry or deprived just to lose weight. I don't make myself hungry in order to keep weight off. I have learned what works for me to make this happen. On the other hand, if I don't get enough to eat, it's not a big deal because I can wait and there will be food later.

There's a difference between being prepared so that I won't allow myself to become EXTREMELY hungry, and eating when I am not hungry just so I won't experience any hunger. You'll have to learn that balance for yourself and what works best for you.

9

Weight Loss Is a Sensitive Subject

Have you ever felt that your life is like a fishbowl when you are on a weight loss journey? Do you feel like people are watching every food decision you make, watching your activity, and noticing if your clothing size is changing?

You might even have people who make it a topic of conversation. Maybe they ask you if you can eat a certain food or if it's on your diet. Did you feel that you had to justify your decisions, or just be quiet and feel bad about yourself?

> *I found power in learning how to be real and honest with the right people.*

Have you found that talking about your weight or about how you feel regarding the weight loss process is one of the "off-limits" parts of your life? I did. I found power in learning how to be real and honest with the right people.

You could be one conversation away from making a big difference in your journey. Consider finding one person that you know, like, and trust. Perhaps that person can be a friend or a professional who will listen to you and not try to fix you. Once you identify that person, consider going through parts of the book together.

My friends and family were concerned about my weight, but they didn't know how to bring it up with me. Even though my husband and I talked about pretty much everything else, I found it difficult to be real with him in this area of my life.

The only time that I would talk about this very sensitive issue would be when I would discuss my latest diet. I kept the talk very surface-level. Anything deeper was off-limits.

Julie Hadden from The Biggest Loser has lost weight and kept it off. She shares about her experience on the Home Word Program:

> She didn't feel that she could trust people in her life with the struggle that she was having with her weight. She never felt that she could be honest with anyone. She was just as miserable with her weight as everyone else in her family.
>
> Some of the things that she would do to avoid having to talk about her struggle with her weight were:
> - She would act as if she was happy to be overweight saying, "Who cares, I like to eat" and chuckle.
> - She became defensive to people they brought it up, "You are just saying I'm not good enough."
> - She would also try to use humor to deflect remarks about her weight. [8]

Some additional ways that people keep this sensitive topic off-limits include:
- Focusing on performance in other areas of life to distract any conversations about weight.
- Blaming someone or something else.

- Giving advice to others about how to lose weight or how to fix their situation.
- Taking care of someone else's needs.

 **Activity 9.1**

Write your answer or talk to someone about your answer.

1. Is there anything that you do to keep from talking about how you really feel about your weight or the process of losing weight?

2. Do you have friends or family members who won't bring up the issue of your weight, or who are insensitive, even if they mean well?

I don't know about you, but I cringe when I hear someone trying to suggest a weight loss solution. They are probably just really excited to share what finally worked for them when other things they had tried in the past hadn't worked. They found the solution to their unique needs and so they want to share that with you. Maybe they know of a solution that other people are using to get results, so they suggest you use that solution because they want you to have the same results.

Many times they don't realize that you might have already tried the very solution they are offering (or something similar) and it didn't work for you. You might even feel worse about yourself because what seemed to work for others didn't work for you. Don't allow that to happen! What works for someone else may not be the solution for you. The program may not work well for you, but you are not a failure.

Maybe you have had people who say things that can be hurtful such as:
- Are you heavier than you have ever been?
- You seem to have a program in place, is this working for you?
- The program is not the problem, it's you.
- You've been doing this program and your results just aren't good enough.

Keep your focus on making one positive and powerful change right now — one that fits you and makes you feel empowered.

Not very helpful, is it? The focus seems to be on the program as the solution and you as the problem. If you have ever felt like that, there is a different way to look at the situation. You just may not have found what works best for you. There is help and you are not a failure just because you haven't had success yet. Don't stop trying!

Try tweaking your own set of solutions. Keep your focus on making one positive and powerful change right now – one that fits you and makes you feel empowered.

 **Activity 9.2**

Discuss with Someone Else

Many times people mean well, but they do not realize that they are not being respectful or empowering in how they talk to someone who struggles with weight.

Things that can seem harmless, actually are not helpful either. For example:
- "You have such a pretty face."
- "Wow, you've lost a ton of weight!"
- "Can you eat that on your diet?"
- Suggesting a program or solution because it worked for someone else.
- Sharing obesity statistics.
- Making fun of someone to try to loosen the conversation, maybe patting the belly.

Questions to consider:

1. What are some other examples?

2. What can those comments mean? How would they make you feel?

3. What are some things that can be said when someone doesn't realize they are not being helpful?

I am grateful that I finally decided to be honest about this area of my life. I was losing weight and I did not want to repeat what happened so many times when I would lose weight in the past and then gain it back later.

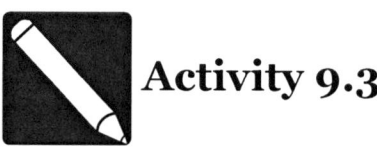 Activity 9.3

Be Real with Someone

- What is it like for you when you receive a compliment about losing weight? Do you like it or dislike it? Why or why not?

- What are you favorite types of compliments to receive? Are there any types of compliments that you would prefer to not receive?

- Have you ever received a compliment that just didn't feel right? If so, what was it? What about when someone describes part of your body when they compliment you, how does that feel? Even if the comment doesn't seem out-of-line, what, if anything, doesn't feel right to you?

- Write down what thoughts go through you mind? Would you prefer people didn't notice? Do you ever find yourself looking for more compliments? Is there anything that you do just because you are looking for a compliment?

In my case, the changes to my body were very noticeable, since many times I would lose as much as 8 clothing sizes. There was so much emphasis on my size. I would receive compliments, even from complete strangers. Most of the time, I truly enjoyed receiving the compliments. It felt wonderful. Yet, receiving the compliments had a dark side to it as well.

I found myself craving the attention because I longed for and needed approval. This type of approval is so easy to get when you are losing weight. I found that becoming smaller tapped into a power and control that is easy for a woman. There was something to the power that came from being able to cause someone to give me a look of approval, even if it was just a glance.

> *I found that becoming smaller tapped into a power and control that is easy for a woman.*

Why would I seek this approval and attention from others when I loved God so deeply and had such a desire to please Him and serve Him?

I am grateful to receive unconditional love from my parents. I have been very happily married, not only once but twice. My first husband, Paul, died of cancer and I am very happy with my current husband, Keith. In both of these marriages, I received plenty of attention and approval. So, why in the world would I have such a longing for this type of attention and approval from others?

What magnified this craving is that I kept it a secret. I didn't feel that I could tell anyone that I thought a lot about seeking attention and approval. It felt shameful to be seeking this type of attention. I found that once I would gain the weight back, I no longer had those looks of approval and it quieted down that craving for compliments from others.

> *I believed a lie and thought that I had "lost my discipline."*

I had no idea at the time that I was intentionally gaining weight. Rather, I believed a lie and thought that I had "lost my discipline" and was falling back into bad habits. Subconsciously, I would just put on weight to stop the attention since people rarely say anything during weight gain. As the weight returned, I would feel protected and my desire for other's approval would decrease.

I had never heard anyone talk about this happening until Dr. Jill Hubbard taught a session at a New Life Ministries [9] event. I learned that I was not the only person who received some benefits of having extra weight. My benefit was to make myself less noticeable. I didn't want to stand out and get extra attention. I wanted to stop my craving for approval. The excess weight made it easier to go around unnoticed. Life seemed less complicated that way.

It helped me greatly to know that I was not alone, many people felt the same way. I hadn't invented my problem and there were solutions that could help me. I had been so ashamed of craving that attention. This went against everything that I valued in my life.

 **Activity 9.4**

Think about some of the "benefits" of carrying extra weight. Write down anything that comes to mind.

I was desperate to make lasting changes in my life. Steve Arterburn of New Life Ministries also helped me greatly with a few simple words. He didn't know any details other than I wasn't particularly comfortable with being a smaller size. Without dismissing how I felt about it, he responded very quickly and told me that I would "get used to it." I felt a sense of relief. Steve normalized my struggle and helped me to see that this is part of the journey and I will be okay. I was not set for that cycle of defeat for life. He took a complex solution and made it simple, which brought me freedom. His words were shared with no judgment or shame, and God used them profoundly in my life.

I have a feeling that most people long to receive approval. I'll be honest, I do still crave approval. I don't ever want to go back to my old ways of trying to get attention in unhealthy ways. So, I continue to be very proactive to protect the gains that I have received.

Thank you so much Dr. Jill and Steve and the whole New Life team. I am glad that God chose you to help me understand what to do with this secret, which had been so powerful in my life. If I had continued to keep this secret, I would never have lost the weight and kept it off. More importantly, I would have stayed stuck in unhealthy patterns that affected many parts of my life.

> ... I would have stayed stuck in unhealthy patterns that affected many parts of my life.

Although it was difficult for me to get to the point of being willing to open up to others, it was worth it to get beyond just surface conversations. The same could be true for you. You just might find out that others feel or think the same way you do.

Points to Consider:

- Get real with yourself and with God.
- Be honest with a friend, support group, counselor or other professional.
- Find someone you can be real with who won't try to "fix" you, yet will speak the truth in love.
- Use discretion as to who you talk to about your weight loss adventure.

- Guard what thoughts go into your mind by choosing wisely what you read and listen to.
- Proactively put into your mind what empowers you on a daily basis.

 **Activity 9.5**

I believed the lie that I had lost my discipline. Write down something that you are listening to that could be a lie.

 **Think about what this verse means to you today.**
Write it down, make a list or sketch it out.
"You will know the truth, and the truth will set you free."
John 8:32 (NLT)

 # Activity 9.6

Have you ever wondered why someone can't or won't lose weight, or why do they do all of that work and then gain it back?

It could have nothing to do with the science or the "how to." It could have nothing to do with the "want to," or lack of willpower or needed discipline. Rather it could be:

- Part of the process was not a fit. Rather than empowering the individual, it backfired.
- The person was missing a tool needed to help sustain the changes.
- Becoming smaller tapped into some things that the person was not ready or equipped to deal with.
- There is a "benefit" of being larger that outweighs the benefits of living at a smaller size.

Tips for you:

- Be careful not to judge the person and assume that they don't care or they don't have the discipline to lose weight.
- Have compassion without feeling sorry for the person, assuming that nothing can be done.
- Don't control or nag.
- Don't enable.
- Ask if there is something that you can do specifically to help.
- Ask if the person would like to share what the struggle is like and just listen without trying to fix the problem.

10

Spiritual Renewal and Empowerment

Lose it for Life puts this well:

"We can, however, pretend to be in control, especially when it comes to losing weight. We pretend by lying to ourselves about the quick fix that fixes nothing or the instant solution that only makes matters worse. We delude ourselves with the mantras of all those who have failed before us:

- All I have to do is have more willpower.
- All I have to do is just stop eating so much.
- All I have to do is quit being so lazy and exercise more.
- All I have to do is take more control of my life.
- I can do anything if I try hard enough.

And when I no longer believe the lie that I can do whatever I set my mind to, I succumb to the opposite extreme, believing I can do nothing and all is hopeless. The murmurs of my aching soul are:

- My weight is genetic and there is nothing I can do about it.
- It's a sin to dig up the past – what's done is done.
- If I was supposed to be thin, I would have been born that way.

We beat our heads against the same brick wall many times before we realize that our own power is not getting us very far."[10]

 **Think about what this verse means to you today.**
Write it down, make a list or sketch it out.
"I once thought these things were valuable, but now I consider them worthless because of what Christ has done. Yes, everything else is worthless when compared with the infinite value of knowing Christ Jesus my Lord. For his sake I have discarded everything else, counting it all as garbage, so that I could gain Christ." **Philippians 3:7-8 (NLT)**

Celebrate Grace

I used to be legalistic, not understanding God's grace. I felt that I really trusted Him and had a close connection with Him. In reality, I only trusted God as long as I felt that I was part of the solution.

That's an awful way to live. I am sure my family would agree that it was unhealthy to live with someone who is controlling and overprotective. I was missing God's grace in many areas of life. My relationship with food was no exception. I really struggled with 1 Corinthians 6:19-20 "Don't you realize that your body is the temple of the Holy Spirit, who lives in you and was given to you by God? You do not belong to yourself, for God bought you with a high price. So you must honor God with your body."

I thought, "If I could be just holy enough, consecrate myself to God, be obedient to Him, then I could lose weight and keep it off." That way of thinking did not serve me well.

Think about what this verse means to you today.
Write it down, make a list or sketch it out.
"... not having a righteousness of my own that comes from the law, but that which is through faith in Christ — the righteousness that comes from God on the basis of faith."
Philippians 3:9(NIV)

I love how Julie Hayden from The Biggest Loser shares this honest prayer "I feel like you are mad at me, God. I am miserable." [11]

God showed her so much about herself. He wasn't mad at her. He was madly in love with her. That reality changed everything for her.

 **Think about what this verse means to you today.**
Write it down, make a list or sketch it out.
"My grace is all you need. My power works best in weakness. So now I am glad to boast about my weaknesses, so that the power of Christ can work through me." **2 Corinthians 12:7-9**

What About Gluttony?

Christian teachings about weight loss can sometimes be based only on Law. This can lead the participants to feel condemnation and shame, even if that is not the intention of the leaders. Sometimes people don't realize how harsh they come across when it comes to eating and losing weight. In my opinion, this only makes the person feel worse about their choices of how much food they eat. Then, it leads to a cycle of shame or trying to fix it on their own.

Overeating and/or gluttony are not talked about in many Christian circles. Just ignoring the issue isn't helpful or empowering. It's important to share truth in a graceful way.

 **Find one or more Bible verses that talk about grace and one or more Bible verses that talk about gluttony.** Write down your thoughts about what these verses mean to you personally today.

Have you found that food is expected, required, or forbidden at social events? Which of these do you find happens often? What if food was no longer any of these things, but was just optional? What could that change?

 **Activity 10:1**

Write down or discuss your answers with others.

1. What is one example of how groups can exhibit grace when talking about weight?

2. What is one example of how someone could come across harsh about food choices or weight?

3. What is one example of how a church overlooks gluttony?

4. What are your choices when you attend events that could tempt you to overeat?

5. What could you do to prevent yourself from overeating at your next event that you attend? Here's some examples that might help:
   - Savor the food.
   - Fill up with water first.
   - Scan for the healthiest choices, making it a priority to eat them first, saving little room for the unhealthy ones.
   - Distract yourself by simply enjoying the company.
   - Eat before or after the event.
   - Have a small serving.
   - Recognize emotional eating patterns even when you are happy or celebrating.

Reality Check

Have you ever been frustrated when a doctor's report was not able to provide a wake-up call for someone you love? I used to spend a lot of time in the doctor's office. In all of those years, only one doctor ever mentioned that my health problems could be related to my weight. I was upset and I dismissed what he had to say.

Another time, I read my doctor's report and I was shocked when I saw that it started off with saying the patient (me) is obese. I thought, "Obese? Surely not!" I was offended. I was not only obese, I was actually close to being morbidly obese. I was quite surprised to learn that someone does not have to be very large to be obese.

> ... an emotional eater is nothing more than someone who uses food in order to change their mood.

This revelation did nothing for me at the time. I did nothing with the information, other than being irritated. Later, I had to quit denying that I had a problem and surrender to God to ask for His help. There were also some things that I had to accept about myself:

- I accepted that I was truly an emotional eater. In the past, I pictured an emotional eater as someone different from me. The truth was that an emotional eater is nothing more than someone who uses food in order to change their mood. It wouldn't really matter what the mood was, the emotion didn't have to be intense. It could be something as simple as being bored and looking for food to help relieve the boredom.
- I accepted that I was an overeater, not just someone with a big

appetite. Previously, I had pictured an overeater as someone who ate more than I thought I was eating at the time.

- I accepted that I needed help and could not fix this problem on my own. I realized that it would take more for me to change than just a diet could provide.
- I accepted that there had to be something different. Losing weight didn't have to be as complicated as I had made it in the past.
- I accepted that getting help was a sign of strength, not weakness.

I did not understand addiction, especially not how addiction would relate to my struggles with losing weight and keeping it off. I denied that I had an addiction. Maybe someone else who was different from me or my circumstances might have an addiction, but not me. I accepted that I was dealing with an addiction.

 **Activity 10:2**

Ask yourself the following questions and write down your answers:
- If I make no changes, what would my life look like in 5 years? 10 years?

- What is not making the necessary changes costing me? What is it costing my family?

- What do I have to gain by making these changes in life? List as many things that you can think of that you would enjoy.

 **Think about what this verse means to you today.**
Write it down, make a list or sketch it out.

"Since we are surrounded by such a huge crowd of witnesses to the life of faith, let us strip off every weight that slows us down, especially the sin that so easily trips us up. And let us run with endurance the race God has set before us."
Hebrews 12:1(NLT)

The Power of Surrender

Surrender is a very important step when it comes to living a life of freedom. Surrender is not being passive. It's actively confessing the need for help and reaching out for that help.

I encourage you to:

- Admit that you need help. You have tried it on your own and you have not been able to accomplish anything lasting or permanent.
- Acknowledge that simply going on a diet won't be enough. If using a food plan works well for you, go with that. Please don't think that's all that you need to do. This doesn't mean that it has to be a complicated process. Pick one thing from the book that you are

willing to do. Get help and move forward with one change at a time.
- Be real with yourself. Do you really want to do the work to make the change, only to have to repeat the process later?

> *You can be a change maker and help people you love to live in freedom.*

You have an opportunity right now to make a difference for the people you care about. There's much more at stake than how much you weigh. The people you love are watching what you do and may follow your example. Please hear me without shame or condemnation. You can be a change maker and help people you love to live in freedom. The change starts with you surrendering to God and working with Him and others to make the changes necessary. There is hope because, with God, all things are possible.

Creating an Environment For Success In the Home

Many of us have specific foods that are harder for us to eat in small amounts. Have you found it helpful to keep those foods out of your home? A popular weight-loss reality show goes into people's homes to see what the family dynamics are like. It's not unusual to see people eating their family member's trigger foods. They often don't realize how they can be sabotaging the success of the person who struggles with food.

Sometimes, family members will complain about having to remove certain foods from the home just because one family member is struggling with it. They feel that they are being deprived to not have whatever food they want in their homes. There have been family members who laughed when they were confronted about bringing certain foods into the home. They just didn't see why it was any big deal.

It's not about depriving family members, rather it's about the family realizing that this is a struggle for the person trying to make changes, and having certain types of food in the home is not always realistic when it comes to breaking a food addiction. It is important to create an environment for success in the home and it takes a willingness to sacrifice for others as well as showing one another respect even if they don't fully understand the process.

> There's only one person who has the right to make the ultimate decision as to what to do with your body, what you eat, and how active you are.
>
> That person is you.

Personal Responsibility

I am personally responsible for what I eat and what I do not eat. No one else is responsible. This includes eating out and going to social events. There's only one person who has the right to make the ultimate decision as to what you do with your body, what you eat, and how active you are. That person is you.

 # Activity 10:3

Imagine that you are with someone who would like for you to eat and you don't want to eat at the moment. Write down one thing that you can say to that person and practice it.

Here are a few ideas:

- "I'm not hungry now, maybe later."
- "I really want to just enjoy your company."
- "I appreciate it. I feel loved just by being with you."
- Chuckle and say, "yeah I want it but I don't..."
- "I'm just so stuffed I can't eat another bite."
- "It looks wonderful, but I think I'll pass for now. But thanks!" Then a really big smile.
- "Can I take some home with me?" Then share it with someone else, eat it, or throw it away.
- "Oh, no, thanks. I already ate."
- "That's so kind of you, but I brought my own food."

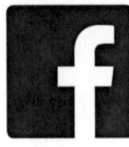 ***Let's Connect:*** Stop in at facebook.com/marylouhelps and share what you can say to someone who would like for you to eat and you don't want to at the moment.

Your next step for taking personal responsibility could be to get help for what you are not able to do on your own. That is a very powerful step.

Character Development

Changing how you relate to food can be an incredible way to develop your character. You may become:

- More courageous
- More considerate
- Better at waiting
- Less controlling
- More perseverant
- A person of higher integrity
- More trustworthy
- More reliable and much more.

 **Think about what this verse means to you today.**
Write it down, make a list or sketch it out.

"Take on an entirely new way of life — a God-fashioned life, a life renewed from the inside and working itself into your conduct as God accurately reproduces his character in you."

Ephesians 4:24 (The Message)

In the past, I was able to lose weight, but I really didn't have much to show when it came to developing my character. When I did my work from the "inside-out," I grew in character.

It took me a while to lose weight for a variety of reasons. I developed some serious health problems and was on medication that caused rapid weight gain and made it very difficult for me to lose weight. Later, extended times of inactivity due to injuries, surgeries and recoveries added to the struggle. I was even able to lose or keep off weight during the times of inactivity because I didn't eat any more than my body needed.

> When I did my work from the "inside-out," I grew in character.

I am now grateful that it was very hard and very slow for me to lose weight. I learned and grew so much more than I ever would have if the weight had come off quickly.

One of the reasons that I was overweight was because I was not good at waiting. I wanted everything "yesterday." This time around, I gained a priceless gift: I can wait now!

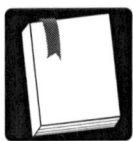

"So let it grow, for when your endurance is fully developed, you will be strong in character and ready for anything."
James 1:4 NLT

 **Activity 10:4**

Name ONE character trait that you feel God is calling you to work on today? Write it down.

From Victim To Survivor To Overcomer

As I would lose weight, I could not help but notice the innocent and not so innocent looks and glances I received. These triggered nightmares and flashbacks of past abuse. I had been an innocent victim and I knew that I needed help. I no longer wanted to live this way. I was in a very dark place in my life to the point that I was barely leaving my home. I was in so much bondage and felt there was no hope. Being overweight was not the cause of my isolation, rather, the isolation lead to weight gain.

> *I had to let go of what worked for others and intentionally embrace what worked for me.*

Dramatic change can happen for anyone. You are not an exception, no matter what. This time, though, it wasn't as complicated as when I tried to fix this part of my life without some very valuable things: I surrendered to God and admitted that I could not do this on my own and needed his help. I also reached out for help from other people. I had to let go of what worked for others and intentionally embrace what worked for me.

It did take work on my part, and therapy also helped. It wasn't always easy, but, I am so GRATEFUL that I didn't have to leave my family, go onto a reality TV show and be weighed wearing just my underwear.

Think about what this verse means to you today.
Write it down, make a list or sketch it out.
"Despite all these things, overwhelming victory is ours through Christ, who loved us." **Romans 8:37**

I have a high respect for the Christian recording artist, Mandisa. I appreciate how she shares that we don't have to wait to be overcomers someday but we are overcomers RIGHT NOW! She was asked in an interview what being an overcomer means to her personally. Here is what she shared:

> "The world is well acquainted with my weight-loss journey – weight-loss and sometimes gain, it's a journey, so it has its ups and downs. I decided to proclaim it for myself. I am not going to be an overcomer once I get to that elusive goal weight. I am an overcomer now.
>
> I love that God makes it really clear that we are not an overcomer because of what we have done. We are an overcomer because HE is an overcomer. He says that in John 16:33 and if

He lives inside of us, 1 John 5 tells us that we are overcomers automatically.

It's easy to base it on circumstances and feelings, but really we are an overcomer because it is in the Word of God and that makes it a fact." [12] – Mandisa

 *"I have told you all this so that you may have peace in me. Here on earth you will have many trials and sorrows. But take heart, because I have overcome the world."* **John 16:33 (NLT)**

We as Christians are overcomers here and now because Jesus is the Ultimate Overcomer.

Read this verse as a prayer by changing words to make them a prayer for your own life. Then write down your thoughts.

"When I think of all this, I fall to my knees and pray to the Father, the Creator of everything in heaven and on earth. I pray that from his glorious, unlimited resources he will empower you with inner strength through his Spirit. Then Christ will make his home in your hearts as you trust in him. Your roots will grow down into God's love and keep you strong. And may you have the power to understand, as all God's people should, how wide, how long, how high, and how deep his love is. May you experience the love of Christ, though it is too great to understand fully. Then you will be made complete with all the fullness of life and power that comes from God.

Now all glory to God, who is able, through his mighty power at work within us, to accomplish infinitely more than we might ask or think." **Ephesians 3:14-20**

Grief

I have been incredibly blessed to have two loving and supportive husbands. I've also experienced great loss in this area of my life when my first husband, Paul, was diagnosed with cancer when we were only 30 years old. Everything in my life was in an upheaval with that diagnosis.

We were very much in love with each other and we loved our young daughters. His cancer treatment was very rough, including all of the chaos that came with battling the disease and trying to be there for the girls. Food offered temporary comfort from the stress and grief during those very rough years.

After 2 years of treatments, Paul was given a clean bill of health by many doctors. We were excited to get started on our new life. But just as everything started to feel like it was getting back to normal, the cancer came back and spread quickly.

I had so many life and death decisions to make and just wanted to grow old with the love of my life while raising our children together. When it seemed evident that he was not going to live, things completely changed for me as far as food was concerned. I found myself with no appetite and that was new territory for me. It took a long time for me to regain a healthy appetite.

> *Don't be hard on yourself when you use food for comfort. Recognize that as a signal that you need help.*

Today, I choose to celebrate for Paul. I can't even begin to imagine how wonderful Heaven has to be for him. I am grateful that I will get to see him someday. That doesn't mean that I don't feel the pain of losing him, or don't miss him. I do feel the pain of missing him and all that goes along with the painful experiences of having my daughters lose their dad when they were at such a young age. Our family has experienced many losses in life.

My brother Greg told me that he would be there for my girls and be their "Dad" since they didn't have one. A few months after Paul's funeral, Greg was killed in an auto accident, leaving behind his wonderful wife and two small children.

I didn't turn to food for comfort during the pain of losing Paul, then Greg soon after. It was not until much later when the heartbreak and grief "caught up" with me. My eyes were more open to how much my daughters were in pain and grieving from so many losses. I didn't know how to deal with the grief, so I returned to my old friend, food. I found that it provided a quick fix, even though the results were temporary.

> *I didn't know how to deal with the grief, so I returned to my old friend, food.*

While it may be common to seek comfort in food when you are facing a challenge, it is important to recognize that there are other choices you can make even during the toughest of times that will serve you much better in the long run. Don't be hard on yourself when you use food for comfort. Recognize that as a signal that you need help. Talk to someone about it, find a therapist or support group, and don't give up.

Lasting Hope and Victory

If someone would have told me years ago that I would one day live free from food and weight issues and be helping others do the same, I would never have believed it. God took my weakest areas and my biggest struggles, and used them for good, which shows that He can do anything!

God has such a sense of humor and has used my story in a very public way. For much of my life, I regained weight just to keep the attention away from my size. My first time to ever be on any type of video was seen by thousands of people in just a few days. I felt as if I had become suddenly visible with all of the attention.

> *I am so grateful that God used the process of losing weight from the inside-out to bring about the most significant spiritual and personal growth in my life.*

The video[13] was made for our church, Northland, A Church Distributed, in Longwood, Florida.[14] Our church sanctuary has very large screens like a movie theatre. The shots were taken close up, so I was extremely large, which is not the way a girl dreams of seeing herself for the first time on video! So many people were not only hearing me share in a vulnerable way, but also seeing my photos in the video. Although it was difficult, I chose to get as far out of my comfort zone as possible, because I knew that my story could make a difference for others.

I now find it funny that, out of all the circumstances in my life that God chose to make public in this video, He chose gluttony! I am honestly grateful that food is my struggle! I never would have imagined that my struggle with food would become a precious treasure to me.

I've had a love/hate relationship with the process of losing weight. In some ways, it could be thrilling if things were going well. I treated it as a project to finish, and then expected to be done with it. The roller coaster of losing and gaining weight, along with starting to lose weight and giving up quickly, was very frustrating.

> *I choose to live an abundant and joyful life, not based on my circumstances. It is well with my soul.*

I am so grateful that God used the process of losing weight from the inside-out to bring about the most significant spiritual and personal growth in my life.

I am thrilled to now be at peace with food and I love to help others find freedom. It's an incredible honor. To me, peace with food means that can I go anywhere I want and I honestly do not notice if food is there. This is such a radical change from when my life seemed to revolve around food, either thinking about it, eating it, noticing it, or controlling it. I am not the food police. People will sometimes feel the need to apologize to me for their food choices, and I honestly wouldn't have noticed what they were eating if they had not mentioned it.

I don't take the positive changes in my life for granted. I could end up losing what I have gained. Relapse could start with a series of little choices. I know the importance of making daily choices to protect what I have gained. This is a high priority to me.

> ... with God's strength, I can choose to not run from adversity.

My relationship with God continues to grow. We continue to face a variety of painful family crises, many with no quick or easy solutions. It continues to be extremely valuable to choose to say things out loud on purpose. One of my favorite things to say is, "I choose to live an abundant and joyful life, not based on my circumstances. It is well with my soul." The more I say it, the more that I believe it and the more that it comes to my mind when I need that reminder.

If someone would have told me years ago that I would have the courage to face these challenges, I would never have imagined it could be true. My husband, Keith, and I find that saying Bible verses out loud every day together is very powerful.

Habakkuk 1:5 God says, "Watch and be astounded at what I will do. For I am doing something in your own day, something you wouldn't believe even if someone told you about it."

Even though I don't like feeling negative things, I know that with God's strength, I can choose to not run from adversity. It gives me great joy to now find ways to give back out of the abundance that God has given to me.

I am continuing to learn that God is working in my life, whether or not I can see the evidence. I can trust Him, even if He doesn't include me in being part of the solution. I can also choose joy and choose to connect with God for who He is and my relationship with Him, rather than just going to Him for what He can do for me.

Yes, the changes on the outside of me are dramatic. I can even fit into just one leg of a pair of shorts that used to be tight on me. In the past, I never kept the weight off for more than a few weeks, now it has been years! Even with those major changes I've experienced on the outside, the changes in my heart mean so much more to me than any exterior change.

God has turned the ugliness of the pain in my life and given me a story and a platform to encourage others and give them hope that He is truly more powerful than any circumstance they could ever face. What it takes to get there is worth it! God has designed each one of us to thrive and have an abundant life, not based on our circumstances.

I can't believe that I get to live this life now! There is hope because with God all things are possible. Please take the step of courage to do whatever it takes for you to grow and not just live but thrive!

11

Group Discussion

Here's one way to use this book for discussion. I encourage you to be creative and do what works best for you.

4 Sessions:

Before the First Session, have group members read Chapters 1-3 and complete the exercise "Finding Your Why".

Session 1: Chapters 1, 2 and 3

Discuss: An activity for Chapter 2 is to take a minute and picture yourself in the future. You have lost weight, and you have kept it off. You think back to how you lost the weight and _____ is NOT on YOUR list of strategies that you used, yet you still had success.

What things come to mind to fill in the blank? What is one strategy that came to your mind?

Discuss:

1. What comes to your mind when you hear the word "accountability?"

2. What doesn't work for you (such as being given a pat answer, being judged based on your food choices, being asked what you ate, being asked what you weigh, etc.)?

3. What does work well for you (such as someone being direct, not being rushed for an answer, etc)?

Ask: Who would quickly like to share your "why?"

End with a quick word of encouragement and look at the between session homework listed. Next session will be chapters 4, 5 and 6.

Notes

Notes

Session 2: Chapters 4, 5 and 6.

Celebrate: Who would like to share one mini-victory since our last time together?

Discuss: Take turns sharing what stood out to you this week in the reading or action steps.

Reflect: Take a moment and reflect what we discussed today. What was your take-away, or what is empowering to you right now? Write it down.

End with a quick word of encouragement and look at the homework that takes place between sessions. The next session will be chapters 7 and 8.

Notes

Session 3: Chapters 7 and 8

Celebrate: Who would like to share one mini-victory since our last time together?

Discuss: Take turns sharing what stood out to you this week in the reading or action steps.

Reflect: Take a moment and reflect what we discussed today. What was your take-away, or what is empowering to you right now? Write it down.

End with a quick word of encouragement and look at the between session homework listed. Next session will be chapters 9 and 10.

Notes

Session 4: Chapters 9 and 10

Celebrate: Who would like to share one mini victory since our last time together?

Discuss: Take turns sharing what stood out to you this week in the reading or action steps.

Reflect: Take a moment and reflect what we discussed today. What was your take-away, or what is empowering to you right now? Write it down.

Ask: What's your plan of action for your next step?

Notes

Homework to Complete between Sessions:

To maximize your results, it's important to be intentional every day. You will move forward in your progress much faster than if you do homework only a few days a week. You don't have to spend much time each day when you are focused and intentional. What you are working on is likely to come to mind throughout the day.

Spend a few minutes every day:

1. Read part of the reading for the week.

2. Do one of the "action steps." It can be a different one each day, or the same one all week.

3. Remind yourself of your "why."

4. Think through your day as consider what helped you and what held you back and write it down.

Today's mini victories	**Today's minor set backs**

At the end of each week, write down:

1. What stood out to you this week in the reading or action steps?

2. Write down one mini victory.

Be ready to share one or the other with the group, if you desire.

Tips for Groups:

General tips for discussion time:
- Silence can be your friend – allow slight pauses.
- Sharing is optional.
- Do your homework and come prepared.

It's helpful to have some guidelines available for the group to read together each time you meet. For example:
- What is shared in the group stays in the group.
- Stay focused on the concepts in the book.
- Please don't share your weight or how much you want to lose.
- Sharing is optional.
- Only share about your own experiences and do not give advice.

Many times, people don't realize how quickly they give advice to try to fix each other. They think that this is helpful, but, often, it is not. Someone in the group might have already tried that solution and is frustrated because it didn't work for them. Also, the person giving advice misses out on the opportunity to share about themselves, which is much more helpful to everyone in the group.

    Encourage your group that this is common and share that you, as a group, are going to practice not fixing each other.

Refrain from saying things like:"Do this_____" or "People should _____."

This skill takes practice. Be open to hearing from someone in the group a kind reminder if are not keeping the discussion about yourself. Ask yourself these questions about how you respond to someone:
- Am I hurt or disappointed if my suggestion is not used?
- Am I giving a suggestion or advice so that I don't need to listen to how God is nudging me?
- Do I feel that I have the solution that can make a difference for someone else?
- Am I giving a suggestion or advice so that I can distract myself from following through on what I need to do?
- Am I giving a suggestion or advice so that I don't need to be honest about myself?

Options to increase connection:
- Between sessions, contact others in the group. Get together in person, by phone, email, etc.
- Have a way of connection for the entire group – a private online group or email. Individual participation is optional.

What about food choices at social events for group? Here are some ideas:
- Have an activity where food isn't included. Go for a walk, play games, etc.
- Have an activity where food is optional. Anyone who wants to eat may bring their own food.
- Have an activity to enjoy the food without judging it (calling it "good or bad") or making it "center stage" for the event.
- When there's food included, plan your social so that part of it does

not include food for anyone who wants to come for the social and not the food.

Tips for Group Leaders:
- Pray for each session, for each person. Ask God to help the conversation to be healthy and helpful.
- Start on time, end on time.
- Start with a quick greeting and possibly a brief prayer.
- Make sure the discussion stays on track.
- Larger groups should be divided into 3-6 women only or men only.
- Silence can be your friend – allow slight pauses.
- Sharing is optional. Rather than going around the room in any particular order, encourage people to share as they are ready.

It's helpful to have some guidelines available for the group to read together each time you meet. For example:
- What is shared in the group stays in the group.
- Stay focused on the concepts in the book.
- Please don't share your weight or how much you want to lose.
- Sharing is optional.
- Only share about your own experiences and do not give advice.

Optional:

You could have a variety of people in the group be in charge of different things, such as starting and ending on time, keeping the group focused, addressing needs of group members between sessions, or any social activities you might add, just to name a few.

Conclusion

God's grace is free. There is nothing you or I could do to earn or deserve it. God loves you unconditionally. Losing weight will not cause God to love you any more than He does right now. If you never change, He still loves you regardless. His love is not based on your performance. What a powerful truth!

> *I never would have imagined that my struggle with food would become a precious treasure to me.*

Finally finding peace with food does not mean that I now have more favor with God than anyone else. I am an ordinary person and grateful for His Grace! His grace is a gift not based on your performance.

I never would have imagined that my struggle with food would become a precious treasure to me. God used the process of losing weight from the inside-out to bring about the most significant spiritual and personal growth in my life. There are so many people who would love to live free from food or weight issues. Some are discouraged and possibly even lost hope that lasting change is ever possible.

I am sharing my story and the things that I have learned in order to encourage you. I don't want you to have to take as much time as I did to find what could make a difference for you. Now, go back to one of the chapters in the book and start there. It does not matter what order you go through the book, start today where you are willing. Read the chapter of your choice and do one of the activities. It is important to be intentional in this effort, and you might even want to set a specific time on your calendar to do the work. It's also important to be honest with yourself and with God. When you are ready, find someone to talk to about your struggle and your journey. Make sure that you choose someone you can be honest with, someone who will listen to you and not try to "fix" you. I promise you, it will be worth it. No matter what your circumstances, there is hope for you, because, with God, all things are possible. Please take the step of courage to do whatever it takes for you to grow, and not just live, but thrive!

References

[1] Cloud, H. (2012, December). *The secret to making New Year resolutions stick.* Retrieved from http://www.foxnews.com/opinion/2012/12/29/secret-to-making-new-year-resolutions-stick/

[2] Brown, B. (2010, June). *Vulnerability.* Retrieved from http://www.ted.com/talks/brene_brown_on_vulnerability.html

[3] Bain, D. (n.d.). Food mood. Retrieved from http://www.calmclass.com/audioPage.html

[4] Dobson, J. (02013, August). *Interview with Allison Bottke.* Retrieved from http://www.drjamesdobson.org/Broadcasts/Broadcast?i=8b75518d-506d-486e-ba34-a1fbd431e501

[5] Mintle, L. (2009). *Press pause before you eat: Say good-bye to mindless eating and hello to the joys of eating.* Howard Books.

[6] Ibid

[7] Ibid

[8] Home Word (2011, April). *Biggest loser gained worth.* Retrieved from https://www.homeword.com/biggest-loser-gained-worth-part-rb-a-1494.html

[9] Newlife (n.d.). Retrieved from www.newlife.com

[10] Arterburn, S. and Mintle, L. (2004). *Lose it for life.* Integrity Publishers.

[11] Homeword (2011, April). *Biggest loser gained worth*. Retrieved from https://www.homeword.com/biggest-loser-gained-worth-part-rb-a-1494.html

[12] Z88.3 radio - Orlando Florida. (2013, August). Sierra Allmand.

[13] Mary Lou Caskey (n.d.). Retrieved from http://www.maryloucaskey.com/media

[14] Northland Church (n.d.). Retrieved from http://northlandchurch.net

Notes

Notes

Notes

Notes

Notes

Notes

Notes

Notes

Notes

Notes

Notes

Notes

Notes

Notes

Notes

Notes

Notes

Notes

CPSIA information can be obtained
at www.ICGtesting.com
Printed in the USA
FFOW03n0722040114
2917FF